THE OBESITY ANTIDOTE

The Path to a Healthier Future: Unveiling the Obesity Antidote

By

Dr Buford. L. Brown

I0696515

Copyright © by Dr Buford. L. Brown 2023. All rights reserved. Before this document is duplicated or reproduced in any manner, the publisher's consent must be gained. Therefore, the contents within can neither be stored electronically, transferred, nor kept in a database. IsNeither in Part or full can the document be copied, scanned, faxed, or retained without approval from the publisher or creator

Table of contents

Introduction

A world where fast food and sedentary lifestyles have become the norm, the battle against obesity rages on. But fear not, for within the pages of this culinary masterpiece, you are about to embark on a transformative journey that will not only tantalize your taste buds but also revolutionize your approach to food and health. Welcome to "The Obesity Antidote," a culinary opus that serves as a beacon of hope in the sea of dietary confusion.

As you open the cover of this remarkable tome, you will be transported into a realm where every ingredient, every recipe, and every culinary creation is a deliberate step toward a healthier, more vibrant life. With the precision of a surgeon and the artistry of a master chef, this cookbook unveils a symphony of flavors that harmonize with the principles of nutrition, balance, and indulgence in equal measure.

"The Obesity Antidote" is not just a collection of recipes; it is a manifesto for a better, more wholesome existence. It transcends the confines of traditional cookbooks, offering you not only mouthwatering dishes but also a comprehensive education on the intricacies of nutrition and the science behind food's impact on our bodies.

Within these pages, you will embark on an epicurean adventure that spans the globe, with recipes inspired by the rich traditions of Mediterranean cuisine, the spice-infused delights of Asian fare, and the comforting classics of home cooking. Yet, each dish is crafted with a singular purpose – to empower you on your quest for a healthier, happier you.

Prepare to be guided by culinary luminaries, renowned nutritionists, and wellness experts who have collaborated to bring you a collection of recipes that are as delicious as they are nourishing. From the exotic and tantalizing to the familiar and comforting, each recipe is a testament to the idea that healthy eating need not be devoid of flavor, joy, or indulgence.

But "The Obesity Antidote" is not just about what you put on your plate. It delves deep into the heart of mindful eating, teaching you how to savor each bite, appreciate the journey of your food from farm to table, and, most importantly, how to foster a loving relationship with your body through nourishment.

Prepare to embark on a transformative culinary expedition. "The Obesity Antidote" is not just a cookbook; it is your passport to a life of vitality, well-being, and the profound realization that taking charge of your health can be a sumptuous, joyful experience. So, turn the page, pick up your apron, and let the healing power of food guide you on a journey towards a healthier, happier you.

Book Description

In a society where unhealthy eating habits and sedentary lifestyles have become the norm, "The Obesity Antidote" emerges as a beacon of hope, guiding you towards a healthier, happier life. This groundbreaking cookbook is not just a collection of recipes; it's a life-changing journey that promises to reshape your relationship with food and help you shed those extra pounds, once and for all.

Why should you purchase "The Obesity Antidote"?

1. Science Meets Flavor: This cookbook is meticulously crafted by a team of renowned nutritionists and expert chefs, combining the latest scientific research with culinary artistry. Every recipe is designed to tantalize your taste buds while nurturing your body.

2. Recipes for All Palates: Whether you're a die-hard carnivore, a devoted vegetarian, or a flexitarian looking for balance, "The Obesity Antidote" offers a wide range of mouthwatering recipes to suit every palate and dietary preference.

3. Empowerment through Knowledge: Beyond recipes, this book educates you about the science of nutrition and the role it plays in weight management. You'll understand

how different foods affect your body and gain insights into portion control and mindful eating.

4. Lifestyle Transformation: Discover the secrets to breaking free from unhealthy habits and building a sustainable, healthy lifestyle. From meal planning to stress management, this book covers it all.

5. Real-World Success Stories: Hear from individuals who have already embarked on their obesity antidote journey using this cookbook. Their inspiring stories and transformations will motivate you to take action.

Family-Friendly: Worried about pleasing picky eaters or getting your family on board? "The Obesity Antidote" includes family-friendly recipes that even kids will love. Say goodbye to mealtime battles.

6. Ingredient Accessibility: You won't need to hunt down rare, expensive ingredients. This cookbook focuses on everyday, readily available items, making healthy eating accessible to everyone.

7. Tools for Long-Term Success: Unlike fad diets, "The Obesity Antidote" equips you with the tools and knowledge needed for lasting success. You'll develop a healthier relationship with food that extends far beyond this book.

8. Community and Support: When you purchase "The Obesity Antidote," you're not just getting a cookbook; you're joining a community of like-minded individuals on a journey to better health. Share your experiences, seek advice, and celebrate victories together.

9. Invest in Yourself: Your health is the most precious asset you have. By investing in "The Obesity Antidote," you're making an investment in your future, ensuring a life filled with vitality, confidence, and joy.

So, are you ready to take the first step towards a healthier, happier you? "The Obesity Antidote" is more than just a cookbook; it's your ultimate guide to transforming your life, one delicious meal at a time. Don't miss this opportunity to reclaim your health and vitality. Order your copy today and embark on a journey to a brighter, healthier future. Your body will thank you, and your taste buds will rejoice! □□□

Chapter One

What is Obesity

Obesity is a complex and multifaceted medical condition characterised by an excessive accumulation of body fat to the extent that it adversely affects an individual's health and overall well-being. It is a global health issue of epidemic proportions, with significant implications for both individuals and society as a whole.

At its core, obesity is the result of an energy imbalance, where the intake of calories through food and beverages exceeds the energy expenditure through physical activity and metabolism. This surplus energy is stored in the form of adipose tissue, commonly known as body fat. While obesity is often measured using the body mass index (BMI), which is a ratio of weight to height, it's essential to recognize that this metric doesn't account for variations in body composition, genetics, and other factors influencing an individual's health.

Obesity can be classified into different categories based on BMI, with severe obesity (BMI over 40) being associated with the most significant health risks. However, beyond BMI, factors like the distribution of fat in the body and the presence of other health conditions, such as high blood pressure, diabetes, and heart disease, play crucial roles in assessing the overall impact of obesity on health.

The causes of obesity are multifactorial and include a combination of genetic, environmental, behavioral, and metabolic factors. Genetic predisposition can make some individuals more susceptible to weight gain, while environmental factors, such as easy access to high-calorie, low-nutrient foods, and sedentary lifestyles, contribute to the development of obesity in many cases.

Obesity is not merely a matter of appearance; it has far-reaching consequences for health. It increases the risk of various chronic conditions, including type 2 diabetes, cardiovascular diseases, certain cancers, sleep apnea, osteoarthritis, and psychological issues like depression and anxiety. Additionally, obesity places a substantial economic burden on healthcare systems due to increased medical costs associated with treating related diseases and conditions.

Efforts to combat obesity involve a combination of lifestyle modifications, including adopting a balanced diet and increasing physical activity. In some cases, medical interventions like prescription medications or bariatric surgery may be necessary. However, preventing obesity in the first place is the most effective approach, emphasising the importance of education, policy changes, and creating environments that support healthy eating and active living.

In cother words, obesity is a complex and pervasive health challenge that goes beyond mere weight gain. It represents a significant public health concern with widespread consequences for individuals and society. Addressing obesity requires a comprehensive approach, including education, lifestyle changes, and policy initiatives to promote healthier living and reduce its prevalence.

Chapter Two

Causes of Obesity Epidemic

The obesity epidemic, a global health crisis that has escalated over the past few decades, can be attributed to a complex interplay of various factors. To comprehensively understand this phenomenon, we must delve into the multifaceted causes that contribute to the rising prevalence of obesity. Here, we shall explore and elaborate on some of the primary drivers behind this epidemic:

1. **Dietary Habits:** Perhaps one of the most significant contributors to obesity is the shift in dietary habits. Modern societies have seen a surge in the consumption of high-calorie, low-nutrient foods, often referred to as "junk food" or "fast food." These foods are typically rich in sugars, unhealthy fats, and additives, making them readily available and affordable, which encourages their overconsumption.

2. **Sedentary Lifestyle:** The advancement of technology has led to a significant reduction in physical activity levels. The prevalence of desk jobs, long commutes, and the proliferation of

screen-based entertainment has resulted in a sedentary lifestyle for many individuals. A lack of regular physical activity contributes to excess weight gain.

3. Marketing and Advertising:

The marketing and advertising strategies employed by the food industry play a pivotal role in shaping consumer choices. Aggressive marketing of sugary and high-calorie products, often targeted at children and adolescents, influences food preferences and consumption patterns.

4. Urbanisation:

The rapid urbanisation witnessed in recent decades has transformed living environments. Urban areas tend to promote sedentary behaviors due to limited green spaces, long commutes, and reliance on automobiles. Additionally, urban areas may have limited access to affordable, nutritious food, pushing residents towards unhealthy options.

5. **Stress and Mental Health:** The increasing prevalence of chronic stress, anxiety, and depression has been linked to overeating and weight gain. Stress can trigger emotional eating and cravings for comfort foods, which are often high in calories and low in nutritional value.

6. **Lack of Education:** Limited nutritional education and awareness can lead to poor dietary choices. Without a fundamental understanding of the importance of balanced nutrition, individuals may inadvertently consume excess calories and unhealthy foods.

7. **Genetics and Biology:** Genetic predisposition can also play a role in obesity. Some individuals may have a genetic makeup that makes it more challenging for them to maintain a healthy weight, even with lifestyle modifications.

8. **Economic Disparities:** Socioeconomic factors contribute significantly to obesity rates. Lower-income populations often have limited access to fresh, nutritious foods and face economic barriers to engaging in physical activities, leading to a higher risk of obesity.

9. Environmental Factors:

Environmental factors, such as the availability of unhealthy food options in neighbourhoods, the design of cities and towns, and the accessibility of parks and recreational areas, can influence obesity rates within communities.

10. Peer and Family Influence:

Social factors also contribute to obesity. Friends and family members often share similar lifestyles and eating habits, which can perpetuate unhealthy behaviours.

Chapter Three

Viral Infections and Obesity

Obesity, a global health epidemic of unprecedented proportions, has captured the attention of researchers, healthcare professionals, and policymakers alike. As we delve into the intricate web of factors contributing to this burgeoning crisis, it becomes evident that obesity is not solely the result of excess calorie consumption and a sedentary lifestyle. It is a multifaceted condition with numerous underlying causes, one of which has gained increasing recognition in recent years – viral infections.

In our quest to understand the complex interplay between viral infections and obesity, we must first recognize that viruses, while primarily known for causing various illnesses, can exert profound and lasting effects on the human body. This chapter delves into the intricate mechanisms through which viral infections can influence the development and progression of obesity, shedding light on a lesser-known yet critical aspect of this global health concern.

The Virogenic Pathways to Obesity

1. **Inflammation as a Culprit:** Many viral infections trigger an inflammatory response within the body, a process aimed at combating the invading pathogens. However, chronic inflammation can disrupt metabolic processes and lead to insulin resistance, a hallmark of obesity.

2. **Virally Induced Changes in Gut Microbiota:** Emerging research suggests that certain viruses can alter the composition of the gut microbiota, influencing how the body metabolises food. These alterations may promote weight gain and obesity.

3. **Neurological Impact: Some** viruses have the ability to infect the central nervous system, affecting areas of the brain responsible for appetite regulation. This can lead to increased food intake and, subsequently, weight gain.

4. **Hormonal Disruption:** Viruses can disrupt the delicate balance of hormones in the body. For example, the human adenovirus-36 has been linked to increased fat accumulation and a higher risk of obesity through its impact on adipose tissue.

The Bidirectional Relationship

Understanding the relationship between viral infections and obesity is not a one-sided affair. Obesity, in turn, can increase the susceptibility to certain viral infections and exacerbate their effects. For instance, individuals with obesity often have weakened immune systems, making them more vulnerable to various pathogens.

Furthermore, the excess adipose tissue in obese individuals can serve as a reservoir for some viruses, allowing them to persist in the body for extended periods. This persistence can lead to chronic inflammation and metabolic dysfunction, further perpetuating the cycle of obesity.

Viral Origins of Obesity: A Historical Perspective

The concept of viral infections contributing to obesity is not a recent revelation. Historical evidence suggests that the adenovirus, initially discovered in the mid-20th century, may have been one of the first viruses linked to obesity in humans. Over subsequent decades, researchers have uncovered additional viral culprits, reinforcing the notion that obesity is not solely the result of dietary choices and lifestyle.

Implications for Prevention and Treatment

As our understanding of the relationship between viral infections and obesity deepens, it opens up new avenues for prevention and treatment. Vaccination against specific obesity-associated viruses could become a viable strategy to mitigate the risk of obesity. Additionally, antiviral medications and therapies that target the consequences of viral infections on metabolism hold promise as potential interventions.

Chapter Four

beverages

Refined sugar and sweetened beverages have become ubiquitous in our modern diet, but their consumption comes with a plethora of demerits that extend far beyond the realm of taste. These products, often alluring in their sweetness, have been linked to a wide range of health issues, environmental concerns, and social problems. In this extensive exploration, we will delve into the substantial demerits associated with refined sugar and sweetened beverages.

1. **Obesity Epidemic:** Perhaps the most glaring demerit is the contribution of these products to the global obesity epidemic. Refined sugar and sweetened beverages are high in calories but devoid of essential nutrients. Consuming them in excess leads to weight gain and an increased risk of obesity, which in turn elevates the risk of numerous chronic diseases such as type 2 diabetes, heart disease, and certain cancers.

2. **Type 2 Diabetes:** Refined sugar consumption has a direct link to the development of type 2 diabetes. The excessive intake of sugar can lead to insulin resistance, where the body's cells become less responsive

to insulin, resulting in elevated blood sugar levels. Over time, this can progress to full-blown diabetes, a debilitating and expensive chronic condition.

3. **Dental Health:** Sugar is notorious for its detrimental effects on dental health. Sweetened beverages and sugary snacks can lead to tooth decay and cavities. The sugars feed harmful bacteria in the mouth, producing acids that erode tooth enamel, leading to painful dental issues and costly treatments.

4. **Cardiovascular Disease:** Excessive sugar intake is associated with an increased risk of cardiovascular disease. Sweetened beverages, in particular, have been linked to high blood pressure, elevated triglyceride levels, and other risk factors for heart disease. This places a significant burden on healthcare systems worldwide.

5. **Liver Damage:** Refined sugar, especially high-fructose corn syrup found in many sweetened beverages, can be particularly damaging to the liver. Excessive consumption can lead to non-alcoholic fatty liver disease (NAFLD), a condition that can progress to more severe liver problems like cirrhosis.

6. **Cognitive Impairment:** Emerging research suggests that a diet high in sugar may have detrimental effects on cognitive function. Excess sugar consumption has been linked to memory problems, cognitive decline, and an increased risk of conditions such as Alzheimer's disease.

7. **Mood and Mental Health:** The consumption of sugary foods and drinks can lead to fluctuations in blood sugar levels, resulting in mood swings and irritability. Moreover, there is evidence to suggest that high sugar intake may be associated with an increased risk of depression and other mental health disorders.

8. **Environmental Impact**: Beyond the health implications, the production of refined sugar and sweetened beverages has significant environmental consequences. Sugar cane and sugar beet cultivation often involves intensive water use, chemical fertilizers, and deforestation. The carbon footprint of transporting and processing these products is substantial.

9. **Social Issues:** The availability and affordability of sweetened beverages, especially in low-income communities, contribute to social disparities in health. These sugary products are often more accessible than healthier alternatives, exacerbating health inequalities.

10. **Addiction and Overconsumption:** Sugar can be addictive, and the frequent consumption of sweetened beverages can lead to cravings and overconsumption. This addiction-like behaviour can be challenging to overcome, making it difficult for individuals to adopt healthier dietary habits.

Chapter Five

Introduction to Healthy Eating

Understanding the Basics of Nutrition

In today's fast-paced and convenience-driven society, the importance of understanding the fundamentals of nutrition cannot be overstated. Nutrition is the cornerstone of a healthy lifestyle and a critical factor in the prevention of obesity and its associated health challenges. This comprehensive guide will explore the core principles of nutrition, emphasize the significance of a balanced diet, and provide you with a selection of delectable recipes designed to combat obesity.

Foundations of Nutrition

At its core, nutrition is the science of how the human body utilizes food to sustain life and promote growth. It revolves around making informed choices to provide your body with the essential nutrients it requires. These vital nutrients can be categorised into five main groups:

1. Carbohydrates:: These serve as the body's primary energy source and can be found abundantly in foods such as grains, fruits, and vegetables.

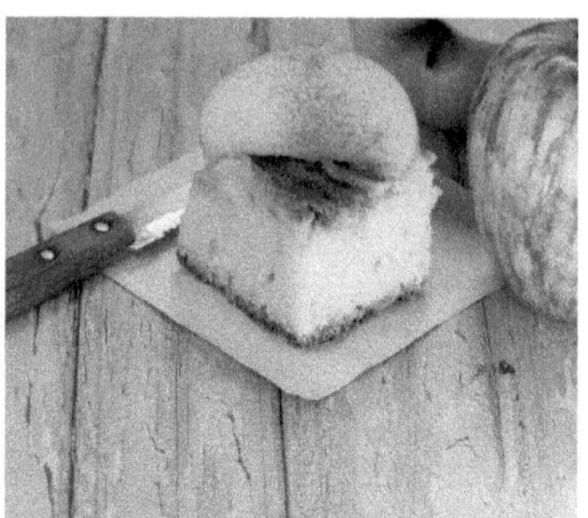

2. Proteins: Essential for muscle repair and overall growth, proteins are prevalent in sources like lean meats, fish,

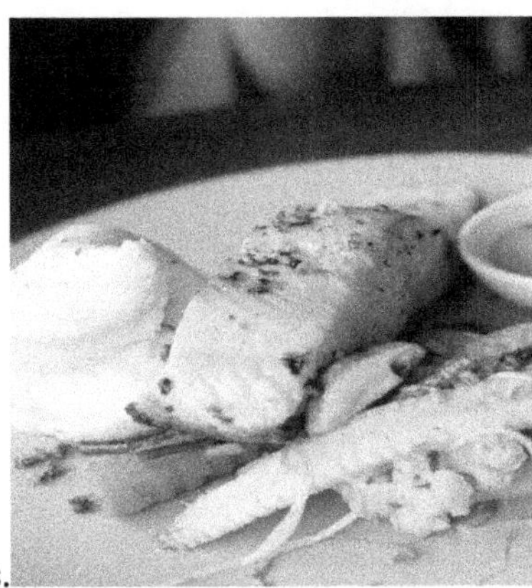

beans, and nuts.

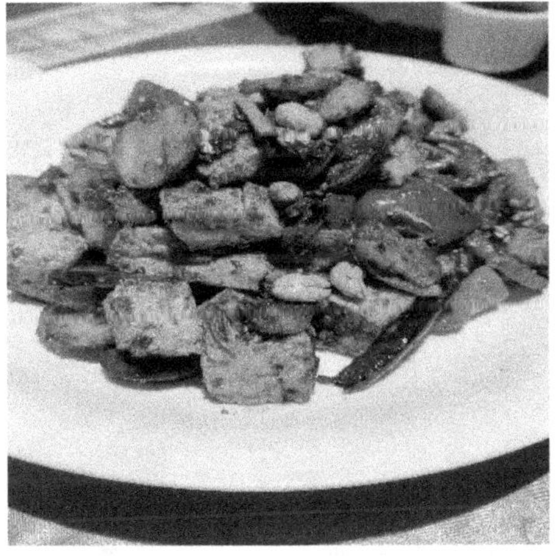

3. Fats: Despite their often-negative reputation, healthy fats are crucial for functions like cell repair and hormone production. They can be sourced from items like avocados, nuts, and olive oil.

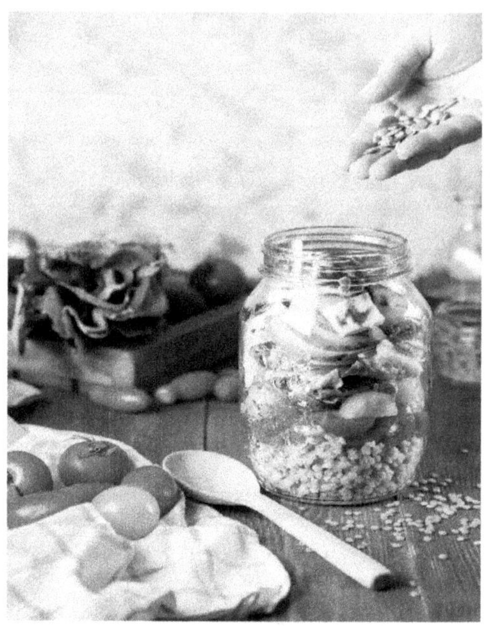

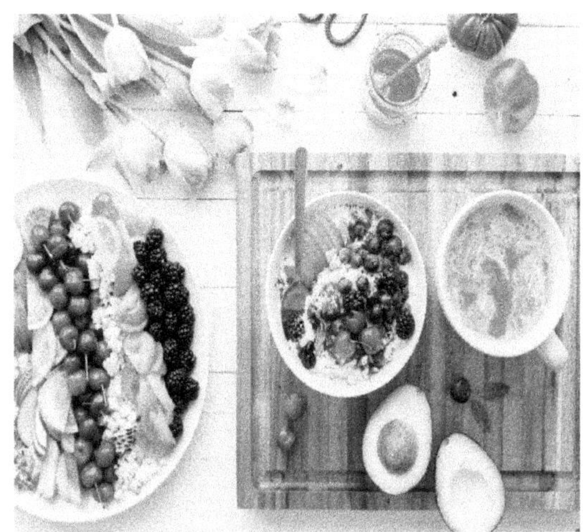

4. Vitamins: These micronutrients play critical roles in various bodily processes and are obtainable through a diverse diet rich in fruits and vegetables.

5. Minerals: Essential minerals like calcium, iron, and potassium are vital for strong bones, oxygen transport, and nerve function, and they can be found in foods like dairy products, red meat, and leafy greens.

The Significance of Balance

A well-balanced diet involves maintaining the correct proportions of these nutrients. Achieving this equilibrium is essential for managing weight effectively and warding off obesity. Here are some key tips to help you achieve dietary balance:

- Portion Control: Mindful portion sizes prevent overconsumption.

- Variety: Diversify your food choices to ensure you receive a full spectrum of nutrients.
- Moderation: Enjoy occasional treats and indulgences in moderation to foster a healthy relationship with food.

Recipes for a Healthier Lifestyle

Now, let's explore some enticing recipes that are not only flavorful but also contribute to weight management:

1. Grilled Chicken Salad: Combine grilled chicken breast with a medley of fresh greens, cherry tomatoes, cucumber, and a light vinaigrette dressing for a low-calorie, protein-rich meal.

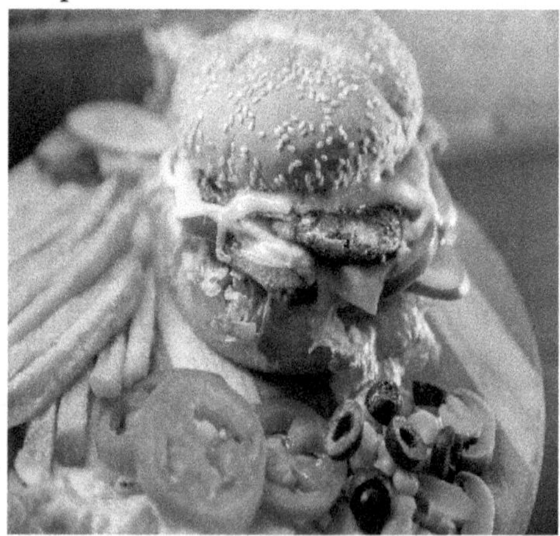

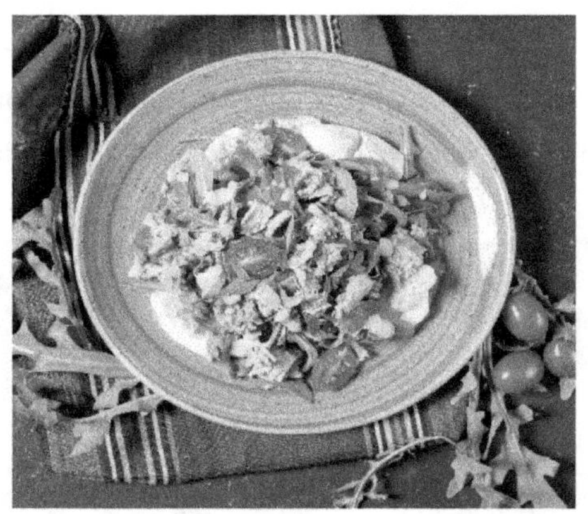

2. Quinoa and Vegetable Stir-Fry: Cook quinoa and stir-fry a colourful assortment of vegetables in a touch of olive oil and soy sauce for a nutrient-dense, satisfying dish.

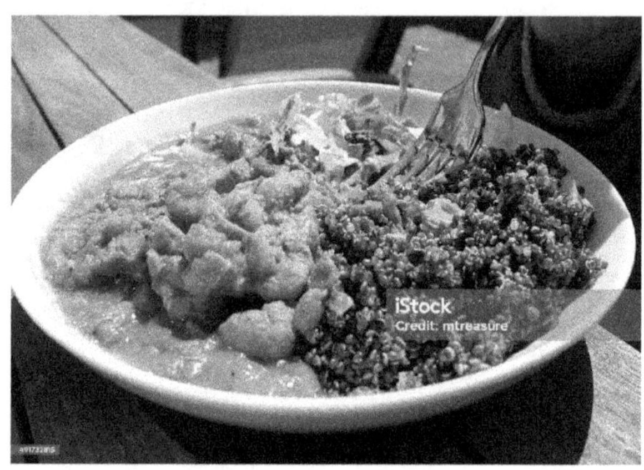

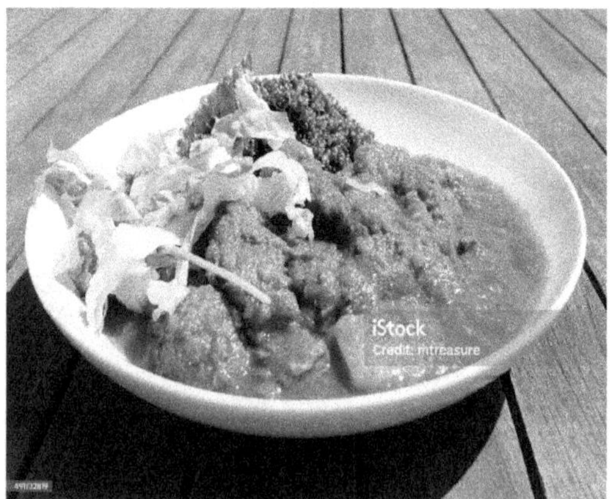

3. Baked Salmon with Lemon and Herbs: Season salmon fillets with herbs and a squeeze of lemon, then bake for a heart-healthy, omega-3-packed option.

4. Greek Yogurt Parfait: Layer Greek yogurt with berries and a sprinkle of granola for a delicious and filling dessert or breakfast choice.

By grasping the fundamentals of nutrition and incorporating these delectable recipes into your diet, you can take significant strides toward preventing obesity and fostering a healthier, more fulfilling life. Keep in mind that healthy eating is not a short-term solution but a lifelong journey toward well-being.

Chapter Six

Breakfast Boosters

The quest for a healthier lifestyle and the pursuit of an obesity-free existence, one cannot underestimate the profound impact of a well-balanced breakfast. This pivotal meal, often referred to as "Breakfast Boosters," is not just a routine task to kickstart your day; it is the cornerstone of optimal health, a powerful tool in the battle against obesity, and the subject of our deep exploration in the pages of "The Obesity Antidote."

1: The Breakfast Revelation

Our journey begins with the Breakfast Revelation, where we delve into the intricate science behind this crucial meal. We uncover how a nutrient-rich breakfast can revitalize your body and mind, setting the stage for a day filled with energy and vitality. From the metabolism-boosting effects to the cognitive enhancements, you'll gain a new appreciation for the transformative power of breakfast.

2: The Obesity Conundrum

As we continue our exploration, we confront the obesity epidemic head-on. "The Obesity Antidote" meticulously examines the factors that contribute to this global crisis. You'll discover the undeniable link between skipping breakfast and weight gain, as well as how Breakfast Boosters can serve as a potent weapon against obesity, fostering a leaner, healthier you.

3: The Nutritional Symphony

This chapter serves as a culinary symphony, composed of carefully selected ingredients that form the Breakfast Boosters ensemble. We unlock the secrets of nutrient-packed fruits, whole grains, lean proteins, and healthy fats, and demonstrate how their harmonious integration can turn an ordinary breakfast into a symphony of health benefits.

4: Crafting the Perfect Breakfast

In the quest to craft the perfect breakfast, we provide a smorgasbord of delicious recipes and meal ideas that cater to various tastes and preferences. From savoury omelettes to mouthwatering smoothie bowls, "The Obesity Antidote" offers an array of culinary delights that will inspire your Breakfast Booster creativity.

5: Maximising the Morning Routine

With a comprehensive understanding of Breakfast Boosters in your arsenal, we pivot towards optimizing your morning routine. Discover effective strategies for incorporating these nutritional powerhouses into your daily life seamlessly, ensuring that you reap their benefits consistently.

6: The Future of Wellness

Our journey culminates in a vision of the future—a world where breakfast is celebrated as the ultimate catalyst for well-being. We explore emerging trends in nutrition, technology, and lifestyle, all geared toward a future where obesity is but a distant memory, thanks to the Breakfast Boosters revolution.

In "The Obesity Antidote," Breakfast Boosters take center stage, showcasing their remarkable potential to transform your health and help you overcome the challenges of obesity. As you turn the pages of this book, prepare to be enlightened, inspired, and empowered to make Breakfast Boosters an integral part of your daily routine. The journey to a healthier, happier you begins with a single, well-balanced breakfast.

Essential Recipes for Breakfast

Energising Oatmeal

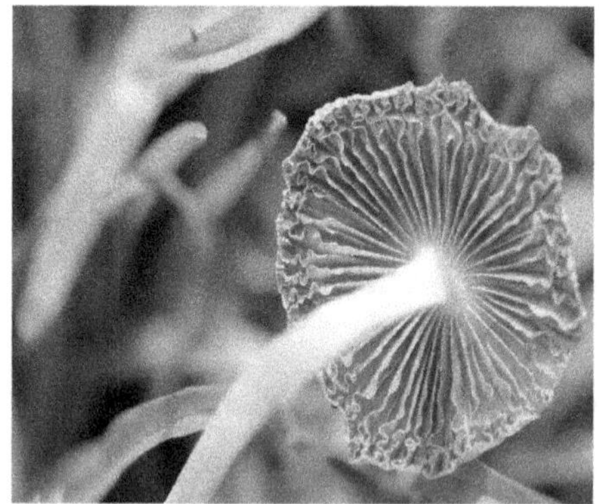

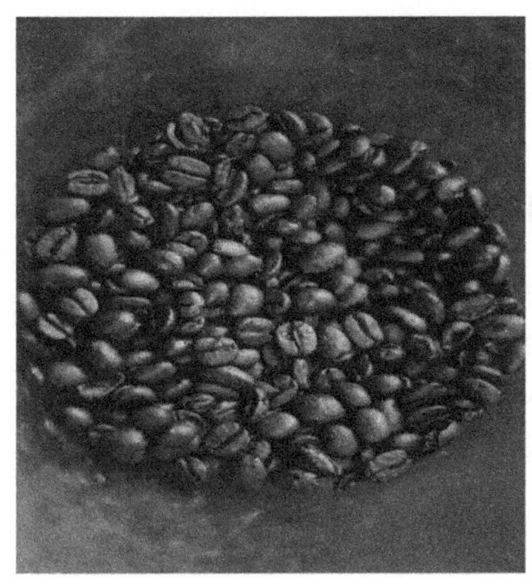

Chapter Seven

When to eat

In the modern world, where sedentary lifestyles and processed foods have become the norm, the importance of mindful eating cannot be overstated. It's not just what you eat, but also when and how you eat that can significantly impact your weight and overall health.

Let's delve into the concept of timing when it comes to eating. Meal timing plays a crucial role in regulating our body's metabolism and energy balance. One of the key aspects of mindful eating is paying attention to your body's hunger and fullness cues. Eating when you're truly hungry and stopping when you're satisfied can help you maintain a healthy weight.

Breakfast, often touted as the most important meal of the day, kickstarts your metabolism and provides the energy you need to start your day. Skipping breakfast can lead to overeating later in the day, as you're more likely to reach for unhealthy snacks to curb your hunger.

Lunch should be a balanced meal that provides you with the nutrients and energy required to sustain you throughout the afternoon. Opt for a combination of lean proteins, whole grains, and plenty of vegetables. Avoid the temptation of fast food or heavy, calorie-laden lunches that can leave you feeling sluggish.

Afternoon snacks, if needed, should be nutritious and portion-controlled. Avoid sugary snacks and opt for options like nuts, yogurt, or fruit. These snacks can help maintain steady blood sugar levels and prevent overeating at dinner.

Dinner, ideally, should be a lighter meal compared to lunch. Consuming a heavy dinner late in the evening can disrupt your sleep and lead to weight gain. Try to finish your dinner at least two to three hours before bedtime to allow for proper digestion.

Furthermore, the way you eat can also impact your risk of obesity. Eating mindfully means savoring each bite, chewing slowly, and paying attention to the flavors and textures of your food. Avoid distractions like watching TV or using your phone while eating, as these can lead to overeating by disconnecting you from your body's satiety signals.

Chapter Eight

What to Eat

In an era where culinary delights beckon from every corner and convenience often trumps nutrition, the battle against obesity has never been more critical. The saying "You are what you eat" holds a profound truth, and by making informed choices about what we put on our plates, we can craft a healthier, more vibrant future for ourselves. Embark on a gastronomic journey with me as we explore a tantalising array of foods that not only nourish the body but also offer the key to avoiding obesity.

1. **Leafy Greens:** The verdant glory of leafy greens like spinach, kale, and Swiss chard cannot be overstated. Packed with vitamins, minerals, and fiber, they provide a sense of fullness while offering a plethora of nutrients, a vital aspect of any anti-obesity diet.

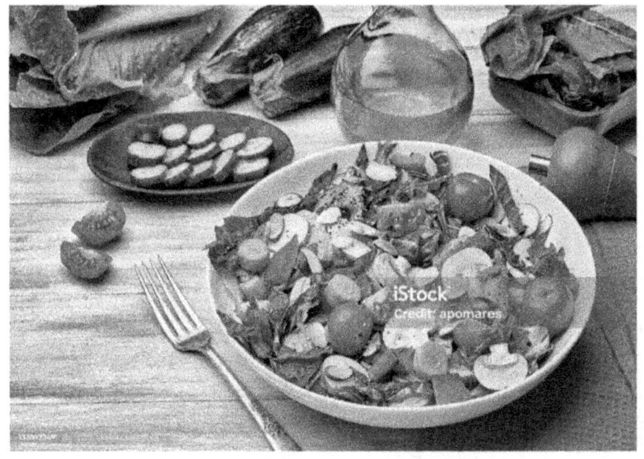

2. **Lean Proteins:** Incorporating lean sources of protein such as skinless poultry, tofu, and fish ensures sustained energy and muscle maintenance. These proteins keep you fuller for longer, reducing the urge to snack on calorie-laden foods.

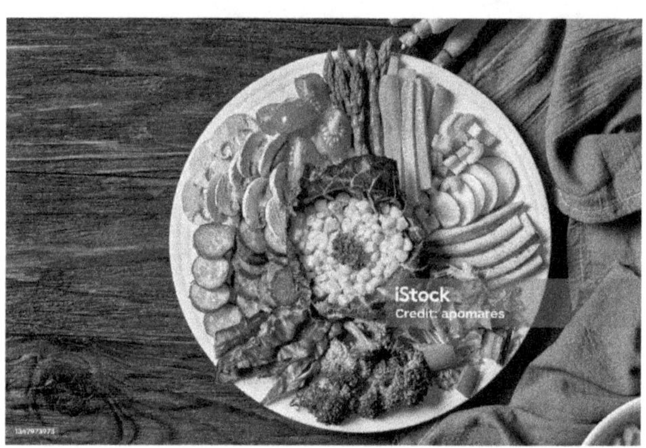

3. Colourful Vegetables: Nature's paintbrush has created an abundance of colourful vegetables like carrots, bell peppers, and tomatoes. They're rich in antioxidants, vitamins, and fibre, making them indispensable for staving off obesity.

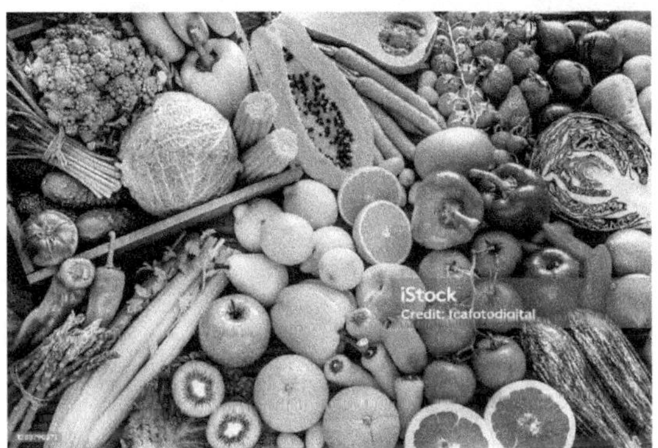

4. Whole Grains: Replace refined grains with whole grains like quinoa, brown rice, and oats. Their high fiber content regulates blood sugar levels and curbs overeating.

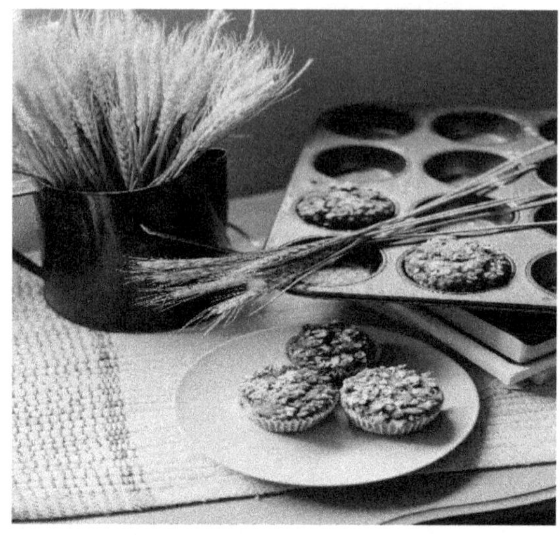

5. Legumes: Beans, lentils, and chickpeas are not just budget-friendly; they are also a powerhouse of plant-based protein and fiber, aiding in weight management.

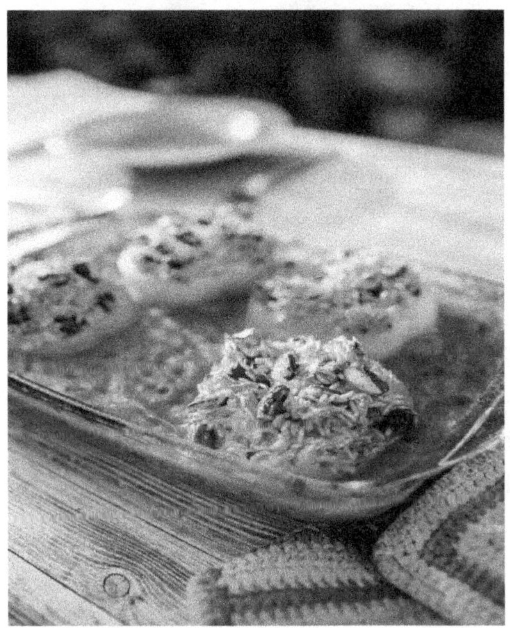

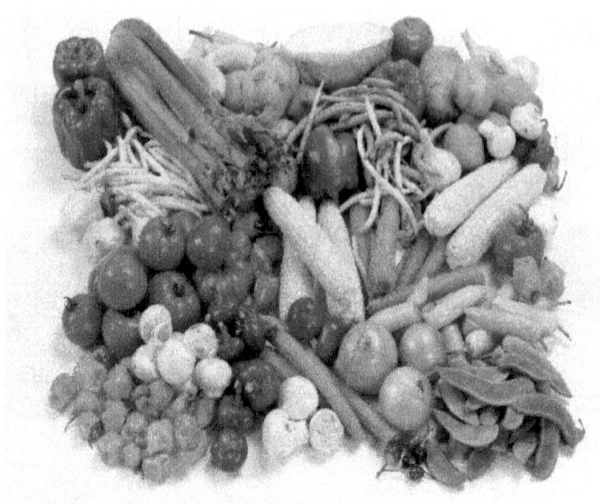

6. Fruits: The natural sweetness of fruits, such as berries, apples, and citrus fruits, satisfies sugar cravings while delivering vitamins and antioxidants that protect against obesity-related health issues.

7. Nuts and Seeds: Almonds, walnuts, flaxseeds, and chia seeds are treasure troves of healthy fats and protein. They provide satiety, preventing mindless snacking on unhealthy fare.

8. Greek Yoghourt: Low in sugar and high in protein, Greek yoghourt supports gut health and promotes a feeling of fullness, making it an excellent choice for those aiming to avoid obesity.

9. Herbs and Spices: Incorporate herbs like basil, oregano, and spices such as cinnamon and turmeric into your meals. They not only enhance flavor but also offer potential metabolic benefits.

10. Water: Often overlooked but crucial, staying hydrated can prevent overeating by curbing false hunger cues. Sometimes, the body confuses thirst with hunger.

11. Portion Control: Regardless of the foods you choose, practising portion control is paramount. Use smaller plates, savour each bite, and listen to your body's hunger cues.

12. Meal Planning: Planning your meals in advance helps you make healthier choices and reduces the temptation to opt for fast food or processed snacks.

13. Mindful Eating: Cultivating mindfulness around food can be a powerful tool. Savor every bite, eat without distractions, and be attuned to your body's signals of hunger and fullness.

14. Regular Exercise: Complementing a balanced diet with regular physical activity is essential for maintaining a healthy weight and preventing obesity.

Chapter Nine

Diet soda delusion

In a quest for healthier choices, diet soda has long been perceived as a savior for those yearning for refreshment without the burden of calories. Its alluring promise of zero calories and guilt-free enjoyment tantalizes the taste buds of millions. Yet, beneath the effervescent surface lies a captivating story of delusion, deception, and the dark side of artificial sweeteners.

Imagine a sweltering summer day, your throat parched, and your desire for a cool, revitalizing beverage intensifying. A diet soda appears as the perfect remedy - bubbles swirling in your glass, offering a taste sensation without the caloric consequences. But here's the unexpected twist: what if I told you that diet soda might not be the virtuous elixir it claims to be?

Enter the realm of diet soda delusions, where perception and reality collide. Many believe that swapping regular soda for its diet sibling is a step toward a healthier lifestyle. After all, it's marketed as a guilt-free pleasure, a way to savor the sweetness of soda without the dreaded calories. But there's a twist in the narrative, as shocking as any plot twist in a gripping novel.

Behind the scenes, diet sodas hide a dark secret: artificial sweeteners. Aspartame, saccharin, sucralose - these sugar substitutes are designed to mimic the sweetness of sugar without the caloric load. However, emerging research suggests that they may not be the magic solution for weight loss and health that we once thought.

The captivating truth is that artificial sweeteners can play tricks on your body and mind. They may disrupt your metabolism, leaving you craving more sugary foods and potentially leading to weight gain over time. Moreover, the alluringly sweet taste of diet soda can dull your taste buds, making healthier, natural foods seem less appealing.

But the story doesn't stop there. Diet soda delusions reach beyond the waistline. Recent studies have linked artificial sweeteners to various health issues, from digestive problems to altered gut microbiomes. These revelations lead us to a captivating question: are we genuinely making a healthier choice when we reach for that seemingly innocent can of diet soda?

In the grand narrative of health and wellness, diet soda's allure can be likened to a mirage in the desert. It beckons with promises of refreshment and satisfaction, but as we draw closer, we realize it's nothing more than an illusion.

Chapter Ten

Fitness and Exercise

Fitness and exercise stand as powerful allies in the ongoing battle against obesity, an issue that has taken on alarming proportions in our modern society. The importance of incorporating physical activity into our daily lives cannot be overstated, and the benefits it brings are nothing short of transformative. In this narrative, we embark on a journey through the world of fitness and exercise, exploring their pivotal roles in combating obesity and enhancing overall well-being.

Obesity, a condition characterized by excessive body fat accumulation, has reached epidemic proportions in many parts of the world. It is not merely a matter of aesthetics but a profound health concern. The consequences of obesity are far-reaching, encompassing a heightened risk of heart disease, diabetes, stroke, and numerous other chronic illnesses. Furthermore, it often exacts a toll on mental health, leading to depression and diminished self-esteem.

However, there is hope on the horizon, and that hope resides in the realm of fitness and exercise. These two elements, when integrated into one's lifestyle, have the power to not only counteract obesity but also to elevate one's quality of life. The journey towards fitness commences with understanding that it is a holistic pursuit encompassing various components: cardiovascular fitness, strength training, flexibility, and balance.

Cardiovascular exercises such as running, cycling, and swimming are exceptional calorie burners, playing a pivotal role in weight management. They elevate heart rate, boost metabolism, and facilitate the shedding of excess pounds. Engaging in such activities not only aids in weight loss but also enhances cardiovascular health, reducing the risk of heart diseases.

Strength training, on the other hand, is the bedrock of a well-rounded fitness routine. It builds lean muscle mass, which, in turn, accelerates metabolism. Resistance exercises like weight lifting, bodyweight exercises, and yoga are indispensable in toning the body and achieving a leaner physique. As muscle mass increases, the body becomes more efficient at burning calories, making it an effective tool in the fight against obesity.

Flexibility and balance exercises may not burn as many calories as cardio or strength training, but they are crucial for preventing injuries and promoting overall well-being. Yoga and Pilates, for instance, improve flexibility, core strength, and balance, thus aiding in maintaining a healthy body weight while reducing the risk of falls and injuries.

Additionally, High-Intensity Interval Training (HIIT) has gained popularity as an efficient method for both burning calories and improving cardiovascular fitness. It involves short bursts of intense exercise followed by brief recovery periods. HIIT workouts are time-efficient and can be adapted to various fitness levels, making them accessible to a broad range of individuals.

Beyond these specific exercises, it's essential to foster a mindset that embraces physical activity as a lifelong commitment rather than a temporary fix. Consistency is key, and finding activities one genuinely enjoys can make the journey to fitness more enjoyable and sustainable. Whether it's dancing, hiking, playing sports, or even gardening, any activity that gets you moving contributes to the overall goal of reducing obesity.

Conclusion

in conclusion, "The Obesity Antidote" serves as a beacon of hope in a world grappling with the growing epidemic of obesity. Through its insightful exploration of nutrition, lifestyle choices, and the profound impact of mindfulness, this book not only offers a comprehensive roadmap to lasting weight management but also invites readers to embark on a transformative journey towards optimal health and well-being.

Dr. Phongsakorn's meticulous research, combined with his compassionate and empathetic approach, paints a vivid picture of the obesity crisis and its deeply rooted causes. With each chapter, he provides a compelling argument for adopting a holistic perspective on health that extends far beyond mere numbers on a scale. It is a call to action, urging us to consider the profound connection between our minds and bodies.

The book's rich tapestry of success stories from individuals who have triumphed over obesity, embracing healthier habits and lifestyles, serves as a testament to the transformative power of the antidote presented within these pages. It reinforces the idea that anyone can overcome the challenges of obesity with dedication and the right knowledge.

In a world inundated with fad diets and quick fixes, "The Obesity Antidote" stands as a steadfast guide, advocating for sustainable change and long-term well-being. Dr. Phongsakorn's holistic approach, blending nutritional wisdom, physical activity, and mental wellness, offers not just an escape from obesity's grasp but a path to a vibrant, fulfilled life.

As we reach the final pages of this remarkable book, we are left with a profound sense of hope, empowerment, and the understanding that true health is within our grasp. "The Obesity Antidote" is not merely a book; it is a lifeline for those seeking a healthier, happier future. It reminds us that the journey to well-being is a deeply personal one, but with the right knowledge and determination, we can indeed conquer obesity and embrace a life filled with vitality and joy. Dr. Phongsakorn's words resonate as a powerful message of change, encouraging us to take that first step towards a healthier, more fulfilling existence.

www.ingramcontent.com/pod-product-compliance
Lightning Source LLC
Chambersburg PA
CBHW061936270726

48660CB00007BA/2804